Organic Shampoos Made Easy

50 DIY Sulfate-Free Natural Homemade Shampoos And Hair Care Recipes For Beautiful Hair

RONNIE ALEXANDER

ISBN-13:978-1512107425

ISBN-10:1512107425

TABLE OF CONTENT

Read Other Books By Ronnie Alexander

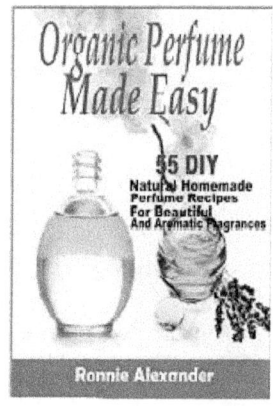

Organic Perfume Made Easy: 55 DIY Natural Homemade Perfume Recipes For Beautiful And Aromatic Fragrances

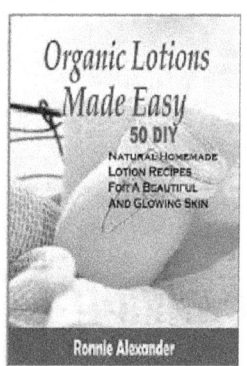

Organic Lotions Made Easy: 50 DIY Natural Homemade Lotion Recipes For A Beautiful And Glowing Ski

INTRODUCTION

Why Homemade Shampoos

Someone may ask 'Why would anyone want to make a shampoo at home when you can buy it from any store?' This question isn't altogether irrelevant. Rather, it is necessitated by the wide variety of shampoos available on the market: shampoos for oily hair, for dry hair, for hair loss, for dyed hair, for curls, for brightness, etc.

There are answers to these questions-And good ones too! Here are a few:

1. **The Ingredients List**

Conventional shampoos contain many harsh and toxic chemicals that may endanger your health. Have you ever bothered to look through the ingredient label on your store-bought shampoo? Many of them contain a plethora of nasty chemicals of which research has proven to cause certain diseases and ailments. Why would you want to put your health at such risk when you can make your own shampoo, enjoy the therapeutic benefits and a lead longer and healthier life while you are at it?

We will come back to listing some of these toxic chemicals that are contained in these shampoos and you will realize how unthinkable it is to spend money on something that may make you sick.

2. **The Cost**

While there are organic shampoos in the market, they are usually expensive. Homemade shampoos will save you a lot of money. The ingredients are readily available and when you buy in bulk, it comes cheaper and last longer.

3. **It's All Fun**

Creating homemade care products is pure fun. It involves combining oils, herbs and foods of all kinds in order to get something perfect for your hair. It is an activity that you will find enjoyable. It is relaxing and satisfying.

Toxic Chemicals In Store- Bought Hair Products

Formaldehyde

This is a chemical preservative used in cheap shampoos. When used, this carcinogenic substance penetrates quickly into the scalp. Prolong usage leads to allergies, dermatitis, headaches and chronic fatigue. Inhalation is extremely dangerous to the eyes, nose and throat (mucous membranes). It is also used to preserve dead bodies.

Dioxane (ingredients ending in Myreth, Oleth, Laureth, Ceteareth)

This is a strong hormone disruptor. It disrupts the function of the nervous system and may cause miscarriages and birth deformities.

Alkylphenol Ethoxylates (Nonylphenol or Octylphenol)

These substances are used as wetting agents to lower the surface tension of liquids so they can foam and then penetrate solid areas. Extremely toxic to fish, they may be carcinogenic and harmful to human's central nervous system. They are hormone disruptor and can also cause asthma, eczema and skin irritations. This is the reason many alkylphenol ethoxylates are gradually being removed as cosmetic ingredients.

Amilia Laureth (Laureth or Lauryl extensions ingredients)

Sodium Lauryl Sulfate (SLS) is the most used. These are synthetic substances found in most shampoos since they are hard foaming agents. They cause eye and skin irritation, hair loss and allergic reactions like eczema. They are often "disguised" in pseudo-natural substances, by the explanation that they "come from coconut". However, they may be contaminated with large amounts of toxins in the manufacturing process. By interacting with other substances, they form nitrates, which are carcinogens.

Parabens - Methyl/ Propyl/ Butyl/ Ethyl/ Isobutyl

These are synthetic compounds included in almost all categories of cosmetics. Manufacturers use them to inhibit bacterial growth and extend shelf life. They are petrochemicals agents with estrogenic, carcinogenic, allergenic and toxic effect. As a result, they can cause fertility problems and affect fetal development. Studies have shown that, in addition to allergic reactions and skin irritation, these parabens are found in tumor tissues of women facing breast cancer. Therefore, their absorption into the body and accumulation over time can cause cancer.

Our Choice Of Shampoos

Having seen the potential risk of buying and using a regular shampoo, let's now point out what drives us in choosing one shampoo over the other.

We all have different expectations for our hair but many of us do not know the difference between a good shampoo and a bad one. This dilemma is further compounded by the well-developed marketing strategies that manufacturers regularly bombard us with. Generally, however, most people look for a shampoo with a reasonable price that would satisfy their expectations. Others go for expensive shampoos with the erroneous thought that an expensive shampoo will make their hair more glamorous and appealing. So what might be considered an ideal shampoo?

The word shampoo has an Indian origin and it means massage. Any shampoo application should be accompanied by massaging the scalp. Gone are those days when a shampoo's function is to simply clean the hair and scalp. Nowadays, it must meet several other requirements: to brighten, to strengthen and to make the hair voluminous.

Manufacturers have also made people believe through their numerous commercials that all good shampoos foam. If they do not foam, they probably will not clean the hair so well. The truth is that foam has little relevance in chemical composition. Foam results when the molecules of the substance with the cleaning ability gather around air and not hair oils. This creates millions of bubbles. So, all the ads showing people with tons of foam in the head just give consumers the wrong idea that hair can only be well-cleaned when there are large quantities of foam.

On the other hand, too much foam shows you are using too much shampoo. Homemade shampoos are not really meant to foam. In the absence of chemical ingredients, the foam is relatively rare. But you can choose your own smell, according to your mood or your hair's needs. And the best part is that you can use plenty of ingredients, including foods, to prepare your hair wash.

Best Ingredients For Various Hair Types

Below are some of the ingredients used in homemade shampoos:

•   Castile soap (available in many homemade shampoos)

•   Filtered/distilled water

•   Jojoba/grape seed/olive/coconut oil

•   Vitamin E oil

•   Vegetable glycerin

•   Dried herbs

•   Essential oils

•   Eggs

•   Yogurt

•   Fruits: lemon, orange, avocado

•   Vegetables: cucumber

•   Honey

•   Aloe Vera

•   Apple cider vinegar

•   Baking soda

- Corn starch

- Ayurvedic powders

Each ingredient brings tremendous benefits to your hair. Your own part is to find out what is best for you. For example, dried herbs work differently on various hair types. Use the following herbs for different hair types:

Normal Hair: use calendula, basil, nettle, linden flowers, sage or chamomile.

Oily Hair: use horsetail, lavender, lemongrass, peppermint, thyme, burdock root or bay leaf.

Dry Hair: use elder flowers, chamomile, sage, parsley leaves or horsetail.

Scalp Ailments: the best herbs are lavender, chamomile, calendula, oregano, peppermint, thyme and eucalyptus.

Hair Loss: use rosemary, sage, nettle or basil

Use The Following Essential Oils For Certain Hair Types:

Normal Hair: carrot seed, clary sage, geranium, thyme, ylang ylang, rosemary, cedarwood, cypress, lavender or juniper

Oily Hair: lemongrass, bergamot, lemon, cedarwood, thyme, clary sage, tea tree, cypress, eucalyptus, geranium, lavender, orange, peppermint, juniper, rosemary, basil, sage, ylang ylang or chamomile.

<u>Dry Hair</u>: rosemary, carrot seed, geranium, lavender, clary sage, sandalwood, chamomile, ylang ylang, cedarwood, jasmine or orange.

Scalp ailments like dandruff, dermatitis, inflammation or itchiness, use orange, cedarwood, tea tree, cypress, lavender, patchouli, marjoram, chamomile, myrrh, rose, rosemary, ylang ylang, sage, rose, thyme, lemon and clary sage

You can see that most of these ingredients are already available in your kitchen. There is also no need for special equipment. All you need are some bowls (for preparing the herbs infusion) and old containers to store the shampoos.

As you begin to change your hair cleansing habits, you might find the homemade shampoos a bit strange as you are not used to putting herbs and foods on your head. Your scalp and your hair are in the same situation but if you are patient, you will be excited by the results you'll get in no time. And your hair will look amazing.

HOMEMADE SHAMPOO RECIPES FOR ALL HAIR TYPES

Olive Oil Shampoo

Enjoy this smooth shampoo that will nourish your hair and leave it shiny and strong.

Ingredients

1/4 cup olive oil

1 cup Castile soap

1/8 cup honey

Directions

1. Combine all the ingredients in a bottle and shake well, until they are well-mixed.

2. Transfer the shampoo to the container and use.

Coco-Milky Shampoo

This shampoo will leave your hair clean and shiny and easy to comb as well.

1/3 cup Castile soap

1/4 cup coconut milk

20 drops of your favorite essential oil

Directions

1. Mix all the ingredients well, shaking to combine.

2. Use the shampoo within a month.

Essential Oils Shampoo

Using this homemade shampoo will enable you benefit from the therapeutic properties of the essential oils.

Ingredients

1/4 cup coconut milk

1/2 cup Castile soap

2 tbsp coconut oil

1/4 cup honey

1 tbsp Vitamin E oil

20 drops Lavender essential oil

30 drops Wild Orange essential oil

Directions

1. Combine all the ingredients in an old shampoo container.

2. Shake well before each use.

Jojoba Oil Shampoo

Use this homemade shampoo to bring back life to your hair.

Ingredients

1 cup Castile soap

2 tsp jojoba oil

1 cup water

1/8 cup aloe Vera gel

5 drops of your favorite essential oil

Directions

1. Use a lid jar to mix all ingredients.

2. Shake before use.

Raw Honey Shampoo

Raw honey is has amazing therapeutic qualities and it's marvelous for your hair.

1 tbsp raw honey

3 tbsp filtered water

5 drops of your favorite essential oil

Directions

1. Mix all ingredients thoroughly.

2. Apply to hair roots and leave it to work for a few minutes. Rinse well with warm water.

Brewed Tea Shampoo

This shampoo is perfect for a shiny, perfect hair. And the smell is fantastic!

Ingredients

1/2 cup baking soda

1 gallon of brewed tea or water

3 tsp xanthan gum

1/4 cup Castile soap

30 drops essential oil of your choice

Directions

1. Bring the water to a boil and place the tea bags. Let them steep for 10 minutes.

2. Take out the tea bags and add the baking soda.

3. Let the mixture cool.

4. Slowly mix in the xanthan gum.

5. Add the other ingredients and stir well.

6. Use as regular shampoo.

Moisturizing Shampoo

This recipe is extremely easy to prepare and the shampoo will nourish your hair.

Ingredients

3 tsp baking soda

2 tsp lemon juice

2 eggs

2 tsp olive oil

Directions

1. Beat the eggs.

2. Mix in all the other ingredients.

3. Apply on the hair and scalp and massage with gentle moves.

4. Rinse with warm water.

HOMEMADE SHAMPOO RECIPES FOR NORMAL HAIR

Oily Herbal Shampoo

The herbs combination will make your hair look amazing, without treating it with harsh chemicals.

Ingredients

2 tbsp dried herbs (combine lavender, linden flowers, parsley leaf, sage)

10 drops Chamomile essential oil

10 drops Geranium essential oil

10 drops Juniper essential oil

10 drops Sandalwood essential oil

8 oz water

1/4 tsp olive oil

3 oz Castile soap

Directions

1. Infuse the dried herbs: simply pour hot water over them, cover with a lid and let steep for at least 5 hours.

2. Remove the herbs and combine the liquid with the other ingredients.

3. Shake well before each use.

Cognac Shampoo

Ever imagined that this drink can be used for hair care? It really does wonders for normal hair.

Ingredients

1 small glass of cognac

1 tbsp honey

1/2 cup organic baby shampoo

Directions

1. Apply as a regular shampoo.

2. Leave it on the hair for 5-7 minutes.

3. Rinse with warm water.

Shiny Lemon Shampoo

You won't believe how shiny and glamorous your hair will look like after using this shampoo.

Ingredients

1/4 cup Castile soap

1/4 cup distilled water

2 tbsp sweet almond oil

2 tbsp dried rosemary

1/2 tsp Lemon essential oil

Directions

1. Infuse the herbs by pouring hot water over them. Leave it until the liquid is a little bit warm.

2. Strain it and combine with the other ingredients.

3. Shake well before each use.

Apple Cider Vinegar & Lemon Shampoo

This homemade shampoo is just right for transiting from regular to homemade shampoos.

Ingredients

2 tbsp fresh lemon juice

1 egg

1 oz olive oil

1 tsp apple cider vinegar

Directions

1. Combine all the ingredients using a food processor.

2. Mix well until smooth.

3. Use as a regular shampoo and rinse well.

Orange & Egg Shampoo

This all natural shampoo will leave your hair soft and shiny.

Ingredients

4 tbsp fresh orange juice

1 egg

Directions

1. Mix these two ingredients until smooth.

2. Apply as your regular shampoo.

Indian Herbal Shampoo

Have you ever noticed the splendid hair of Indian women? They all use the same hair care routine with herbs and natural oils.

Ingredients

17 oz shikakai

9 oz Greem Gram/mung beans

9 oz fenugreek

3 oz soap nuts

1 package basil/tulsi leaves

1 package curry leaves

Directions

1. Leave your ingredients to dry in the sunlight for at least 12 hours.

2. Transform into a powder by grinding them.

3. Store in a jar.

4. Each time you want to use your herbal shampoo, take a small amount, mix it with water until you form a paste and apply to wet hair.

Peppermint Shampoo

Boost your senses with this refreshing homemade shampoo.

Ingredients

1/4 cup Castile soap

2 tsp jojoba oil

1/4 cup distilled water

1/8 tsp Tea Tree essential oil

1/8 tsp Peppermint essential oil

Directions

1. Combine all the ingredients and leave the distilled water to the end.

2. Shake well before use.

HOMEMADE SHAMPOO RECIPES FOR DANDRUFF

Easy Essential Oil Shampoo

The essential oils in this shampoo will softly remove the dandruff from your hair.

Ingredients

1/4 cup Castile soap

1/8 cup honey

1/8 cup coconut

1/2 tbsp Vitamin E oil

1 tbsp coconut oil

5 drops Lemon essential oil

5 drops Lavender essential oil

5 drops Carmella essential oil

5 drops Rosemary essential oil

Directions

1. Mix all ingredients in a jar.

2. Use within a month.

Natural Herbal Shampoo

Get rid of nasty dandruffs with the help of natural herbs.

Ingredients

1.5 oz Castile soap

4 oz water

1 tbsp dried herbs (Calendar, Chamomile, Oregano and Nettle)

1/8 tsp olive oil

5 drops Cedarwood essential oil

5 drops Cypress essential oil

5 drops Tea Tree essential oil

5 drops Rosemary essential oil

Directions

1. Pour hot water over the dried herbs and let them infuse for at least 4 hours.

2. Strain the liquid and combine it with the other ingredients.

3. Shake well before each use.

Jojoba Oil Shampoo

The combination of natural oil with apple cider vinegar will help you fight the dandruff.

Ingredients

1/4 cup Castile soap

1/4 cup distilled water

1/2 cup jojoba oil

3 tbsp fresh apple juice

1 tbsp apple cider vinegar

6 garlic cloves, minced

Directions

1. Use a food processor to mix all the ingredients.

2. Turn it on low until the mixture is smooth.

3. Use as a regular shampoo.

Sweet Honey Shampoo

Take advantage of the therapeutic properties of honey and let it nourish your hair.

Ingredients

6 tbsp warm water

2 tbsp raw honey

10 drops of your favorite essential oil

Directions

1. Let the honey melt in the warm water. Add the essential oil.

2. Use as your regular shampoo.

Black Soap Shampoo
All the ingredients from this excellent shampoo will help your scalp fight dandruff.

Ingredients

1 cup hot water

4 tbsp African black soap, crumbled

3 tbsp grape seed oil

2 tbsp raw honey

Directions

1. Combine all the ingredients and mix well.

2. Allow to cool before you apply on your hair.

Lemon, Honey & Egg Shampoo
This shampoo will remove the dandruff from your hair and will leave it clean and shiny.

Ingredients

2 eggs

3 tbsp fresh lemon juice

1 tbsp raw honey

3 drops olive oil

Directions

1. Beat the eggs. Combine the lemon juice and the honey.

2. Mix in the eggs and add the olive oil.

3. Apply on hair. Rinse with warm water.4.

Aloe Vera & Essential Oils Recipe
Fight dandruff with this recipe.

Ingredients

1/2 cup Castile soap

2 tbsp aloe Vera gel

1/2 tsp vegetable glycerin

2 drops Lavender essential oil

5 drops Tea Tree essential oil

2 drops Rosemary essential oil

Directions

1. Mix all the ingredients well.

2. Use as regular shampoo and remember to shake before use.

HOMEMADE SHAMPOO RECIPES FOR HAIR LOSS/GROWTH

Quality Hair Loss Shampoo

If you have problems with hair loss, then you need to try this homemade shampoo.

Ingredients

1/4 cup honey

1/4 cup coconut milk

1/2 cup liquid Castile soap

1 tbsp Vitamin E oil

2 tbsp coconut oil

10 drops Rosemary essential oil

10 drops Cedarwood essential oil

10 drops Peppermint essential oil

10 drops Lavender essential oil

Directions

1. Combine all the ingredients in a bottle with a lid.

2. Shake well before use.

All Herbs Shampoo

The combination of herbs will strengthen your hair and will help it regenerate.

Ingredients

8 oz water

2 tbsp dried herbs (combine rosemary, sage, nettle and basil)

3 oz liquid Castile soap

1/4 tsp jojoba oil

10 drops Cypress essential oil

10 drops Ylang Ylang essential oil

10 drops Lemon essential oil

10 drops Peppermint essential oil

Directions

1. Let the herbs infuse for at least 5 hours after pouring hot water over them.

2. Remove them by straining and then combine the liquid with all the other ingredients.

3. Shake well before each use as the ingredients tend to separate.

Soap Nuts Shampoo

Ayurvedic plants (reetha &shikakai) have been used by centuries for hair care. This shampoo is excellent for hair growth.

Ingredients

2 tsp shikakai powder

3 oz soap nuts/reetha

Directions

1. Leave the soap nuts to soak overnight in a bowl.

2. Transfer all the content to a food processor.

3. Add the shikakai powder. Mix well.

Lemon & Amla Shampoo

Amla is well known amongst Indian women. It is used for hair growth.

Ingredients

1.5 oz Amla powder

4 tbsp fresh lemon juice

Directions

1. Form a paste from these 2 ingredients.

2. Apply to wet hair.

3. Rinse well with warm water.

Glycerin Shampoo

Ingredients

The vegetable glycerin will nurture your hair, regenerating it and making it strong and healthy.

1/2 cup organic shampoo

1/2 tsp vegetable glycerin

2 tbsp aloe Vera gel

1 capsule Vitamin E

3 drops Peppermint essential oil

5 drops Rosemary essential oil

2 drops Bay essential oil

Directions

1. Combine all the ingredients and mix well.

2. Use as regular shampoo.

Reetha, Amla & Shikakai Shampoo

These 3 ayurvedic herbs have been used for centuries to improve the quality of hair and keep it healthy and strong.

Ingredients

1 tbsp Reetha powder

1 tbsp Shikakai powder

1 tbsp Amla powder

A few tbsp of warm water

Directions

1. Combine the three powders.

2. Slowly pour the water until you get a spreadable paste.

3. Apply to the damp hair and leave it on for 15 minutes.

4. Rinse well with warm water.

HOMEMADE SHAMPOO RECIPES FOR OILY HAIR

Herbal Glossy Shampoo

Use this herbal shampoo to balance your oily scalp so that your hair becomes clean and shiny.

Ingredients

3 oz liquid Castile soap

8 oz water

10 drops Bergamot essential oil

10 drops Clary Sage essential oil

10 drops Geranium essential oil

10 drops Rosemary essential oil

2 tbsp dried herbs (use a combination of calendula, chamomile, nettle and thyme)

Directions

1. Infuse the herbs for at least 4 hours (pour hot water over them).

2. Remove the herbs by straining them and then place the liquid into a bottle.

3. Add the other ingredients and mix well.

4. Shake well before every use.

Baking Soda Super Duper

Try this super easy recipe to remove the excess sebum from your hair.

Ingredients

1 cup warm water

1 tbsp baking soda

Directions

1. Prepare a solution by mixing the two ingredients.

2. First, massage the hair roots. Secondly, apply the solution to the hair length.

3. Rinse well using warm water.

Green Clay Shampoo

Green clay is well known for its detoxifying properties and the fact that it helps regain the oil balance of the skin and scalp.

Ingredients

1 tbsp Castile soap

1 tbsp green clay

10 drops tea tree oil

2 tsp green tea

Directions

1. Mix all ingredients. Use as your regular shampoo.

2. Rinse with warm water.

Aloe Vera Cleansing Shampoo

Combine the soothing properties of aloe Vera with the cleansing qualities of lemon and you will get the perfect shampoo.

Ingredients

2 tbsp fresh lemon juice

1 tsp aloe Vera gel

1/2 cup Castile soap

Directions

1. Combine all the ingredients and mix well.

2. Use as a regular shampoo.

Avocado Fatty Shampoo

Although avocado is rich in fats, it helps the scalp restore its natural oil balance and removes the grease from the hair roots.

Ingredients

2 tsp baking soda

1 ripe avocado, mashed

1/4 cup warm distilled water

Directions

1. Mix all ingredients.

2. Apply to wet hair. Let it stay for 5 minutes and then rinse with warm water.

Glycerin & Essential Oils Shampoo

The mix between the essential oils and glycerin will establish the natural oil balance for your hair.

Ingredients

1/2 tsp vegetable glycerin

1/2 cup Castile soap

4 drops Juniper essential oil

1 drop Cedarwood essential oil

5 drops Rosemary essential oil

Directions

1. Combine all the ingredients.

2. Shake well before use.

HOMEMADE SHAMPOO RECIPES FOR DRY/FRAGILE HAIR

Therapeutic Shampoo
Use the therapeutic power of essential oils to strengthen your hair.

Ingredients

1/2 cup honey

1 cup liquid Castile soap

4 tbsp coconut oil

1/2 cup coconut milk

2 tbsp Vitamin E oil

30 drops Lavender essential oil

30 drops Wild Orange essential oil

40 drops Clary sage essential oil

Directions

1. Use an old shampoo container to place all the ingredients.

2. Shake well to combine.

3. Use within a month.

Dry ABC Shampoo

This shampoo is very easy to prepare and will help your fragile Hair

Ingredients

2 tbsp rice flour

2 tbsp arrowroot powder

2 tbsp cornstarch

10 drops Lavender/Lemon essential oil

Directions

1. Mix all the ingredients until well incorporated.

2. Place the mixture to the hair roots using your hands.

3. Brush to distribute the shampoo all over your hair.

4. You don't need to rinse it.

Lemon/ Cucu Shampoo
For Fragile Hair/Dry Scalp

Ingredients

1 lemon

1 cucumber

Directions

1. Peel the two ingredients.

2. Use a food processor to mix them together.

3. Apply the paste as your regular shampoo.

4. Rinse thoroughly and be mindful of the tiny lemon parts that tend to remain in the hair.

Apple Cider Vinegar Shampoo
Instead of spending your money on expensive hair treatments, use this all natural shampoo for your dry hair.

2 tbsp apple cider vinegar

1 cup Castile soap

1/4 cup water

1 tbsp Tea Tree oil

Directions

1. Combine all the ingredients and mix them well.

2. Use as your regular shampoo.

Coconut Milk Shampoo

Use the powerful moisturizing properties of coconut to take care of your dry hair.

Ingredients

1/4 cup coconut milk

1 tbsp sweet almond oil

1/3 cup mild organic shampoo

10 drops of your favorite essential oil

Directions

1. Combine all the ingredients in an old shampoo container.

2. Shake well before use.

Creamy Avocado Oil Shampoo

If you plan on spending your whole summer at the pool, your hair will certainly get dry. Use this natural shampoo to keep its oil balance.

Ingredients

4 oz Castile flakes

1/4 cup avocado oil

1/4 gallon water

Directions

1. Bring the water to a boil and cover the flakes.

2. Mix well until everything is cool.

3. Add the avocado oil and stir until well incorporated.

4. Store in a clean container.

Glycerin Rich Shampoo

This shampoo will nourish your hair and leave it soft and smooth.

Ingredients

1/2 tsp vegetable glycerin

1 drop of Chamomile essential oil

1 drop of Geranium essential oil

1 drop of Ylang Ylang essential oil

1 drop of Clary Sage essential oil

5 drops of Lavender essential oil

1/2 cup organic baby shampoo

1/4 tsp Vitamin E oil

Directions

1. Place all the ingredients together and stir well.

2. Use as regular shampoo.

HAIR CONDITIONERS

Apple Cider Vinegar Conditioner

Keep your hair clean with this homemade conditioner.
Apple vinegar successfully removes all the shampoo traces.

Ingredients

1/2 cup apple cider vinegar

2 cups water

Directions

1. Combine the two ingredients.

2. Shake well before use.

3. Rinse your hair with this mixture and don't worry about the smell: you won't feel it.

Banana Deep Conditioner

This conditioner will leave your hair soft and easy to brush.

Ingredients

2 tbsp raw honey

1 ripe banana

2 tbsp olive oil

Directions

1. Use a blender to mix all the ingredients.

2. Apply the paste to the hair. Let it work for 30 minutes.

3. Rinse well.

Egg & Yogurt Conditioner

Bring a lot of vitamins to your hair by using this egg-based conditioner.

Ingredients

1/2 cup mayonnaise

1 cup plain yogurt

1 egg

Directions

1. Combine all the ingredients.

2. Apply on scalp and hair.

3. Leave on for 40 minutes.

4. Rinse with lukewarm water.

Coconut Oil & Honey Conditioner

Use this extra moisturizing conditioner that combines the richness of honey with the great properties of coconut oil.

Ingredients

2 tbsp honey

3-4 tbsp coconut oil

Directions

1. Place the two ingredients in a bowl and the bowl in a pan half filled with water.

2. Let the coconut oil melt and mix well.

3. Apply the mixture on the scalp and hair and leave on for 30 minutes.

4. Rinse well.

Cinnamon & Milk Conditioner

Use this conditioner to keep your hair stronger and healthier.

Ingredients

2 tbsp honey

2 tbsp cinnamon powder

4 tbsp milk

2 eggs

1/4 cup mayonnaise

Directions

1. Combine all the ingredients in a jar.

2. Place it in bowl with warm water.

3. Apply the heated mixture on hair and scalp. Don't forget to use a shower cap.

4. Leave the conditioner on for 30 minutes.

5. Rinse well.

Avocado & Shea Butter Conditioner

This conditioner is ultra moisturizing and it's just right for those with thick hair.

Ingredients

1/2 cup Shea butter

1 ripe avocado

3 tbsp apple cider vinegar

Directions

1. Use a food processor to mix all the ingredients.

2. Lather the mixture on the scalp and hair.

3. Leave on for 30 minutes.

4. Wash your hair with warm water.

Orange & Yogurt Conditioner

The conditioner will maintain your hair, keeping it shiny and strong.

Ingredients

1/4 cup fresh orange juice

1 cup plain yogurt

1/4 cup coconut milk

4 tbsp lemon juice

1 egg

Directions

1. Combine all the ingredients and mix well.

2. Apply on wet hair and let it stay for 30 minutes.

3. Wash hair with a homemade shampoo.

HOMEMADE SHAMPOO RECIPES FOR COLOR ENHANCERS

Shampoo For Golden Highlights

Keep your hair blond without burning it with harsh chemical substances.

Ingredients

1.5 oz Castile soap

4 oz water

1 tbsp dried Chamomile, Sunflower petals and Calendula

Directions

1. Bring the water to a boil and pour it over the herbs.

2. Allow it to steep for at least 5 hours.

3. Remove the dried plants and combine the liquid with the other ingredients.

Shampoo For Dark Highlights

The herbs from this shampoo will enhance the dark color of your hair.

Ingredients

1 cup homemade shampoo of your choice/organic shampoo

2 tbsp black tea, black walnuts hulls (crushed), comfrey root

8 oz hot water

Directions

1. Infuse the herbs in hot water for at least 5 hours.

2. Remove the plants and combine the liquid with the shampoo.

3. Mix well and use as regular shampoo.

Shampoo For Red Highlights

Use this all natural shampoo to keep the red shades of your hair.

Ingredients

1 cup organic shampoo

2 tbsp henna, hibiscus flowers, red rose petals

8 oz hot water

Directions

1. Cover the herbs with hot water, put a lid on the bowl and leave on for 4 hours.

2. Strain the liquid and combine it with the shampoo.

3. Mix well and use.